SEX MASSAGE TONIGHT:

The Simple, Easy to Read Guide That Will Have You Massaging Your Partner...Tonight

INTRODUCTION

There are many books and guides that teach long, drawn-out massage techniques and methods. That is NOT what this book is about. This book is about giving your partner an awesome erotic massage as soon as possible. You don't need a degree in massage therapy to give your partner something they'll really love. All you need is the desire to give the best massage you can—everything else is easy, and this book with give you a few guidelines, then walk you through a classic sexual massage you can use on your partner as soon as *tonight.*

Now, the only that's better than a regular massage is a SEXUAL and EROTIC massage, deep and sensual—pleasure that comes from the sensation you feel when the flesh is given erotic attention. Of all the organs of your body, your skin is the largest with literally thousands of nerve endings, and the sense of touch has the power to stimulate all of the senses.

Before starting with the massage, there are a few basic guidelines to keep in mind when giving this kind of fantastic pleasure to your partner.

ENVIROMENT

Let's get one thing straight—a sexy massage needs to be in a place where the *mood is right.* First off, make sure the room is clean and straightened (usually the bedroom, but it can be anywhere.) Lighting is very important—keep it dim, because you are going to be lighting candles. Candles are an absolutely essential part of a mind-blowing erotic massage, and should not be overlooked. Try to avoid the scented candles if possible, as incense is much better to burn. Set the mood—light the candles, burn a little incense, make sure it's clean. Take time to make the bed comfortable and soft, and just as crucial as candles is *music.* No heavy rock or DJ music here—find something very soothing to play. Some of the softest and most romantic music can be found for free online on Youtube(.com). Do a search for "432 hz music" and you can find many wonderful ambient and instrumental tracks that run for over an hour. You can also use nature sounds as well, including rainforest, thunder, or waves on the beach, which all work well. We want our partner to be stimulated, not fall asleep, so take a moment and pick something great. Also make sure your music is either on "repeat" or continuous play because the massage time can vary, and once you begin you won't want to stop to adjust your stereo or computer. Turn off all cell phones, lock the door and make sure you silence anything else that could be distracting—keep your pets, if you have any, in another room as well.

OILS

Another key factor in sexual massage is choosing a great massage oil. You can get massage oil most health food stores or spas, and even some grocery stores or pharmacies keep them in stock as well. You can also order many different oils online as well. Find one that is either unscented or mildly scented, and make sure to test a small amount on your partner's skin in the rare case they may be allergic. Try to pick a water-based oil, and additionally try to avoid oils that contain Nonoxynol-9, which can irritate the skin. Keep your oil nearby and within reach because you will need it to maintain optimum lubrication for the smoothest possible massage. Additionally you can choose an "edible oil" for massage on the genitals. Warm the bottle of oil in a bowl of warm water, to get the bottle and oil warmed for your partner. No cold oils!

SKIN CONTACT

Remember when giving the sexual massage you should never break the contact with the skin of your partner. Once you have begun the massage, you will need to maintain the connection with your partner the whole time. Breaking contact dissolves the intimacy quickly and can make the person receiving the massage very uncomfortable. As a side note, check your nails for any sharp edges or hangnails that could be painful for your partner, especially in the erogenous zones.

TAKE YOUR TIME BEING GENEROUS AND BE GENTLE

A very important thing to remember is that there should be no rush when giving your massage. Draw the massage out as long as is appropriate, being generous with your strokes as well as tender and gentle. It's important to keep every movement sensual, which usually means *nice and slow*. A great sexual massage can feel like time is standing still for your partner, so really get into it and enjoy every bit of the process, which can be very rewarding for the one who is giving it. The process is a slow build that increases the tension until it reaches a "breaking point" of sexual desire that will leave you and your partner breathless. So have fun with it, but yes, take your time, and be gentle.

DRINKS

Keep a couple glasses of water nearby for you and your partner. If you're feeling extra romantic make it two glasses of wine or two sweet cups of juice. Have something you can both sip on occasionally if necessary.

USE THE BATHROOM FIRST

This should be fairly obvious, but before you begin both you and your partner should use the bathroom prior to starting. It is optimal if you can find time make sure both of your bowels are emptied, but just making sure you go "#1" will do.

THE SEXUAL MASSAGE

Have your partner first strip down completely nude. Have them lay on the bed or floor face down on a soft, clean blanket. You are going to have to be able to reach any and all parts of their body without any effort. Have a sheet handy to place over your partner's back. It is very sensual when you move down their body during the massage to adjust the sheet down as you work further and further down. Remember, NO part of your partner's body will remain untouched.

Now, begin with your warmed oil by oiling up yourself first. Take off your clothes, (underwear is optional), and spread the oil across your own nude body first, where your partner can watch. You'll be using your hands, but you are going to want your arms and chest greased up nicely. This is an incredible turn-on, so you're already beginning the massage with an erotic gesture that will let your partner know you are serious about their sexual massage. Once you have oiled yourself up, it's your partner's turn.

Take a generous amount of oil into your hands, rubbing them together to warm it. Remember; never directly pour oil onto your partner, always put it in your hands first. Now, with your hands well oiled, start by gliding with long, smooth strokes with the palms of your hands over the shoulders and neck, and up and down the arms. Keep your movements smooth and rhythmic, maintaining contact the entire time.

Work your partner this way for several minutes, paying extra care to the shoulders. In most people, tension is usually stored the most in the shoulders, so take your time in this area and really work them well.

When you have liberally massaged these areas, you can start working your way down the back, making your strokes longer and deeper. This is another area you're going to want to spend some time, but use your body for the pressure, not your arms, and make sure your breathing is relaxed and rhythmic. Eventually you can press your oiled chest against your partner's back, sliding up and down, letting your nipples and other areas lightly graze against their body.

The sensation of skin brushing against skin will be highly stimulating for your partner, especially since you will both be well oiled. Give your partner a kiss on the jaw, then move to her neck, giving it gentle kisses as you work the back softly and slowly. If you chose edible oil, you can lick the lower part of the back in round, circular movements, moving up the body as your breathe lightly with warm breath along the line of the spine until you arrive at the ear lobes, where you can kiss you partner lightly, driving them absolutely wild.

By now, your partner should be past the stage of feeling relaxing and instead be getting **HOT**—you are well on the way. Just make sure you're keeping the contact going, because now you are going to start massaging areas that are even more erotically stimulating.

Next, start to move back down your partner's body where you can massage their buns. Make sure your partner's legs are open where you can lightly graze up and down the inner thighs. If you want to make your partner squirm in delight, remember that touching the inner thighs sensually will cause that exact reaction. It is built into humans naturally and is an involuntary reaction of an area that is easy stimulated into pure pleasure. Still, take time massaging your partner's buns, using the palms of your hands, starting with the right cheek, massaging it firmly yet carefully. When you have worked the right cheek completely, move to the left and repeat. Your partner will feel a stirring in their loins—stimulating the buns can awaken desire in almost anyone!

After you have generously worked the buns, you will roll your partner onto their back, taking care to keep a hand on them as you help them turn over. Do you still have enough oil? If you don't, use a free hand and liberally lubricate your partner's chest. Gently massage their shoulders working down the arms and back up again. Skim over the chest with the palms of your hands, using plenty of warm oil. You can give the chest a few circular movements over your partner's hard, erect nipples. Remember, that massaging the chest is always a prelude to sexual contact. That is why we end with the massaging and stroking of the chest. If we started with the chest, it would be awkward. The chest is *always* last, and is the doorway to the genitals.

Time to take stock—does your partner love it? Listen to their breathing, their sighs—their moans. Your unique sexual chemistry with your partner will let you know when they want more, and by now, their pleasure has certainly turned to outright desire.

After feeling the sensations in the nipples, your partner will be eager for stimulation, this time in their genitals. A woman will be hot and wet, yearning for penetration, and a man will be visibly erect, with the probability his penis will be "twitching," which means it aches for touch. Do you go for these areas right away—sort of, but no quite yet. Remember, we need to take our time, especially now, because there is no turning back and you should really prolong the feelings of desire as much as possible—this will only increase the magnitude of both you and partner's inevitable orgasms. Most likely they will be breathing hard or moaning, and you will want to kiss down their stomach, into their inner thighs.

Position yourself between their legs, bringing a leg up as you kiss the insides of their thigh. Now you will begin massaging their genitalia—but only skimming over lightly. If you are massaging a woman work the lips of the vagina, bringing the middle finger inside to hit her G-spot several times. If you are massaging a man, cup his balls with one hand while delivering broad strokes up and down his cock. For men or women, it is important to start slow and build your strokes. Don't be rough—make every movement sensual and purposeful. No mindless jerking! Each stroke needs to be slow and passionate, continually building. Your partner will be so excited it will be difficult for them to bear. Experiment with your movements, paying close attention to their reactions as to where they seem to enjoy it the most and how what you are doing is working—

when you hear a moan of pleasure, work that spot a little longer. Glide a hand off their genitals and tweak, rub, and tug on their nipples. By returning to this area it will surely magnify their desire off the charts.

By now your partner will surely want and need to experience the pleasure of penetrative sex. Whatever sexual partner you are working with, make sure you ease the penis (or dildo, if you are a lesbian), in just a little, and then out. Nice and slow—do not begin humping furiously. Keep dragging it out. Very, very slowly, allow the penetration to occur little by little. Keep up the teasing.

Once the actual sex is initiated, you'll be taking it from there—read your partner's body language, communicate with them, and enjoy it. When you both reach orgasm (which can happen quite quickly, due to the amazing foreplay that YOU created) your orgasms will be vital and potent, and very, very intense. You will be amazed how sexual massage can take the pleasure to realms you didn't even realize existed.

* * *